CW00839772

Understanding M.E –
A Guide For Friends,
Family & Carers

HAYLEY GREEN

ISBN: 1507646313
ISBN-13: 978-1507646311

DEDICATION

This book is dedicated to Ken, who knew me before I was ill, and was there for me when I was diagnosed.

Thank you for being so patient and understanding, willing to learn about my illness when you didn't know what it was, and for your help throughout. Thank you for the comfort through the tears, the hugs over the years, showing that you care.. and for simply being there.

Thank you to my friends, you know who you are, and my family, for supporting me through this, and believing in me.

CONTENTS

1 What Is M.E?   1

2 Understanding Symptoms   Pg. 7

3 Understanding Limits   Pg. 13

4 How To Help   Pg. 18

5 Facts & Quotes   Pg. 21

1 WHAT IS M.E?

For many people, M.E is not a 'well known' illness. Certainly when I was first diagnosed with it, I didn't really know what it was. Many years ago, it was the same with M.S (Multiple Sclerosis) – and nowadays most people are familiar with the name. Possibly the most frustrating part of having the illness is lack of understanding – from friends, family society and even the medical profession.

So what is M.E?
The name stands for Myalgic Encephalomyelitis. Now that's a mouthful! Let's break it down: Myalgic stands for *Muscle pain and inflammation.* Encephalomyelitis means *Inflammation of the brain and spinal cord* - usually due to a viral infection. To break it down further:

My = Muscle
Algic = Pain
Encepahlo = Relating to the brain
Mye = Relating to the spinal cord
Itis = Inflammation

It is perhaps more commonly known as 'CFS' or 'Chronic Fatigue Syndrome'. This is a term which many suffers prefer not to use. The term implies that the illness is simply 'fatigue' (If only!), however where fatigue can be a prominent symptom it is one of many symptoms that a sufferer may experience. It is a bit like calling Emphysema 'Chronic Coughing Syndrome' – it just doesn't come near to covering all of the symptoms experienced, so most sufferers prefer to use the term M.E. In some countries it is referred to as PVIDS or, Post-viral Immune Dysfunction Syndrome.

So how do people 'get' M.E? In most cases there is a trigger for the illness, very commonly a viral infection. I was diagnosed after a bout of tonsillitis almost four years ago, which I never got better from – this is called a precipitating factor, or in other words, a trigger. There are also predisposing factors which put a person at risk of developing M.E. These can include long term stress, recurrent viral infections or a traumatic experience such as an accident or bereavement.

M.E has been classified as a neurological disorder since 1969, by the WHO (World Health Organisation). Neurological is defined as related to the nervous system. This means that several areas in the body are affected, including the immune, lymphatic, hormonal, cardiovascular and musculoskeletal systems. This is why the disease produces such a wide range of symptoms.

Examples of other neurological disorders are MS and Epilepsy.

To be diagnosed with the illness, a patient needs to be suffering from symptoms for at least 6 months. In most cases a GP will make a diagnosis and then refer the patient to a specialist clinic, or a consultant such as a neurologist or rheumatologist, where confirmation of the diagnosis may be made.

M.E is a fluctuating illness. This means that the severity of symptoms can change over weeks, days, and even hours. A sufferer will never know how they are going to feel on a given day, until they wake up.

A very unique factor separates M.E from many other illnesses. Post-exertional malaise means an increase of symptoms after exertion.

Often with M.E, the effects are not seen until 24-48 hours after the activity. This means that suffers experience 'payback' for everything they do. Sometimes we can do more, but then feel much worse for the next few days. We can get bursts of adrenaline, which allow us to operate above our normal level of activity, but once this wears off, we suffer profusely.

M.E affects approximately 250,000 people in the UK. It is the biggest cause of long term sickness in schools, including both children and teachers – as quoted by Invest In ME.

It is a long term, debilitating illness. Each patient experiences different symptoms and severity of symptoms. Many with the illness are housebound or wheelchair bound, and roughly 25% are severely affected and bedbound. Some affected severely are on oxygen and need to be tube fed. At worst, it can be fatal. It affects people of all ages and backgrounds.

M.E is a physical 'organic' illness, and over 60 outbreaks have been recorded since 1934.

People who have the illness are permanently excluded from donating blood or organs. There is no cure, and treatment is limited to symptomatic relief. The root cause is still unknown, and it receives little government funding.

Charities such as *Invest In ME* campaign for bio-medical research into the cause and treatment.

The prognosis (forecast/outlook) for the illness is variable and very difficult to determine. A small number of people may recover completely – and some find improvement over time, but many get worse. It is often thought that the sooner a person is diagnosed and the illness treated, the more chance there is of a full recovery. However with careful management of the illness, improvement can happen.

It varies from person to person and there is no indication as to when someone may recover. Often people have regular relapses, where the illness will worsen for a period of time, and then improve. Relapses are intermittent, and can be caused by pushing past limits, emotional stress and viral infections amongst a host of other situations. We look at the limits of an M.E sufferer in more detail in chapter three.

So there are the basics! You may be reading this guide because a friend or loved one has been diagnosed with the illness, or you may care for a sufferer and want to understand it better. It's okay not to know what it is – a lot of people don't. What's important is that you are willing to learn and understand, and that quite possibly could be the greatest gift you could give anyone suffering from it.

In my personal experience, I have found the most difficult thing to deal with is the general lack of knowledge and understanding about it. Often when you tell people, they ask 'What's that?'. Trying to find the words to explain it, proves even more difficult.

Even more so is having an 'invisible' illness. Sometimes we don't 'look' ill, but we can be terribly unwell on the inside. Unfortunately pain and fatigue cannot always be seen.

M.E is a recognised disability (a long term condition which affects a person's daily life and activities) under the Equality act.

2 UNDERSTANDING SYMPTOMS

What are the symptoms of M.E? This chapter aims to help you understand many of the more common symptoms we experience.

Fatigue

Fatigue is a feeling of complete and utter physical, mental and emotional exhaustion. Unlike normal tiredness, it cannot be relieved by sleep or rest. No matter how much sleep we get – we always wake up unrefreshed, feeling like we haven't slept. Day in, day out. This alone is extremely debilitating. We simply can't function. The fatigue we experience is the kind you may get after full blown flu. The wiped out, shattered feeling it gives you, where you are barely able to move due to the lack of energy. This is normal for an M.E sufferer, but we get used to it. I can't remember how it feels to have energy. To experience the fatigue that we do, a healthy person would probably have to stay awake for three days straight!

Pain

Pain is another predominant symptom with this illness. Although it cannot be seen, it can have a tremendous effect on our lives. Living with chronic pain is hard. Especially when no one can see it! The aches we feel are comparable to a healthy person running a marathon. Sore all over, feeling 'bruised' and full body aches. This is the type of pain that we have to live with. Often painkillers serve no purpose, and it can make us feel incredibly grumpy or low. Which is quite understandable, if you can imagine being in pain for weeks, months or even years. The best way I can describe the muscle pain is feeling as if you have been beaten all over with a stick! Muscles are tight, knotted and sore to touch. We can injure ourselves very easily – a common occurrence for me is waking up with a pulled muscle... I am pretty sure I don't do gymnastics in my sleep!

Joint pain is another symptom we can get. A dull, intense ache deep down in our joints. If you have arthritis or similar then perhaps you can understand, but the only way I can describe it is that it's like a knife twisting inside of you.

Headaches

Now you've probably all experienced a headache! They linger like a bad smell, and can make you extremely irritable. Imagine daily headaches, ones you wake up with, that may go away – or may stay all day no matter what pain relief you take. It's like having your head in a permanent vice. This is quite normal to experience if you have M.E.

Nausea & Dizziness

The best way to describe this is to liken it to travel sickness. That awful spinning feeling you get, and the intense nausea along with it can be unbearable. Many M.E sufferers have this on a regular basis. Some people may vomit and it's extremely debilitating to live with. Every time you stand up, you feel light headed, sick and dizzy. Every time you move your head, again you feel as if you are on a fairground ride. This can last for hours, days or weeks! Some people pass out regularly.

Post-exertional Malaise

You will often hear an M.E sufferer talk about this. It's our worst enemy! If we push past our limits, then you can guarantee that this will hit us. We pay for everything we do. One day we may feel well enough to go out, or to meet friends etc. – but the next day, we pay for it with a full increase in symptoms. It is tempting to do more when you are feeling a little better, to 'live' a little, but we know that for every high there is a low. We all have different limits, so doing too much for someone suffering mildly could be cooking dinner after going to work. For someone more severely affected, this could be a short phone call. It doesn't have to be a physical task.

Anything that requires mental, physical or emotional energy can drain us. For some, attending a doctor's appointment could means weeks in bed to recover afterwards.

Cognitive Dysfunction

The damned 'brain fog'! Brain fog, you say? This is what we call our cognitive issues. These may include memory problems, word finding difficulty, slurring or stuttering. A foggy brain feels like a brain stuffed with cotton wool. We can put something down, and a few seconds later forget where we have put it. We can be talking and in the middle of a sentence completely forget what we were saying. This can be embarrassing, and we often feel silly. It's what you would expect with dementia, except this isn't – it's a prominent symptom of M.E. Often we will put things in silly places, or forget the smallest of things. Our minds can't process too much information, so looking at a long piece of writing can be very exhausting. People with the illness often find travelling in a car very draining. It's almost like our eyes can't process the road in front of us, and it still working on overdrive trying to take it all in. Your head literally feels like mush. Saying that, I and those around me do find my 'foggy moments' quite amusing!

Flu-like symptoms

Often our immune systems produce symptoms similar to the flu. This is incredibly frustrating, because sometimes you aren't sure whether you are coming down with something, or you are having a 'flare up' of symptoms. Sore throat, shivers, hot sweats and body aches. We tend to get hot sweats most at night time, and have an overall temperature intolerance – either feeling too cold or too warm. So you may often see us shivering, or furiously fanning ourselves!

Sleep Disturbances

It's almost inconceivable to wonder how we can be so fatigued yet sometimes be unable to sleep. Some M.E sufferers experience chronic insomnia. The problem is, we don't feel tired – we feel ill. When you're aching, feeling sick, and feeling very poorly in general, the last thing your body wants to do is sleep. Some people find that their sleep patterns are reversed, some can only sleep for an hour or so at a time and some sleep for most of the day and night, yet still wake up exhausted. Sleep issues are very common for us sufferers and again, can fluctuate over time.

Emotional Issues

Many who have M.E Also have depression, most commonly as a symptom of the illness, or a result of the illness. The two must not be confused! Imagine your whole life changing, going from busy, active and social to housebound or bedbound. I think it's fair to say that this would make anyone feel low. We can experience stress, anxiety and depression as a result of having to live with the illness, and so many M.E sufferers are prescribed anti-depressants to help them cope with the physical symptoms and effects of the illness on day to day life.

These are just a few of the more common symptoms of the illness. Everyone is different and experiences different symptoms. I find that symptoms change over time – I can have several weeks where I have mostly pain, or a few days where I am very dizzy and nauseous. The unpredictability is a source of frustration to many.

Other symptoms that may be experienced are:
- Tremors / shaking
- Fainting
- Seizures
- Stroke or coma like episodes
- Paresthesia
- Heart palpitations
- High heart rate

- Gastrointestinal symptoms (IBS for example)
- Sensitivity to noise, light and sound

.

3 UNDERSTANDING LIMITS

So now you will have a fairly good idea of the symptoms that we may experience. But how do they affect us in our day to day life? This chapter will help you understand our limitations and more about the nature of the illness.

As you will know, the illness fluctuates. This means we often can't make plans ahead. We could arrange to meet on a particular day, wake up that day and feel well enough to be able to socialise. Or we could wake up and not be able to get out of bed. This is why many of us will be hesitant to make plans, because we don't want to let people down. Often people will see us when we are able to have visitors, and go out. We may even appear to be 'ok' – but we are so used to hiding our symptoms it becomes second nature. If we spoke about feeling unwell, we would be saying it all day. Just because we may not talk about our illness doesn't mean we aren't in pain, or fatigued, it's that we are so accustomed to it that over time you become used to feeling like it and putting on a brave face.

There are lots of things you can do once – including jumping off a cliff! We may be able to do something one day, but not the next. This is how our illness fluctuates. It's like a box of cruel tricks, waking up and wondering what symptom it's going to throw at you today. A good way of describing our energy levels (or lack of) is by imagining a battery. A normal healthy person will wake up and feel refreshed with their battery at 100%. This will drain very slowly, so they may go to work, then go for drinks with a friend, come home and cook dinner, bath/shower and then catch up on television.

Those who suffer from M.E will wake up with their 'battery' on red, let's say 30% compared to a healthy person. This 30% has to last all day, and our battery drains at at a much faster rate. So everything we do is chipping away at our energy. Get dressed… that's 5% gone. Make breakfast, another 5%. Have a lay down and you may get that 5% back, so here we are at 25%, and it's not even halfway through the day yet. Have a long telephone conversation, that's another 10% gone. It's not even time for dinner and we are running on 15%. We must use that 15% wisely. Shall I cook? Or shall I have a long bath? I know if I cook that will take me right down to 0%, anything else is into energy reserves that we don't even have, and then we are overdoing it – which means payback tomorrow!

One thing I never envisaged having to do was to make choices about such simple things that I once took for granted. This is what we have to do. For many we have barely enough energy to do the things we have to do, let alone the things that we want to do. It must be frustrating when we can't do something, or have to decline invitations. We may even seem rude and unsociable. But this is the reality we are faced with. You can sure bet we would love to go and have a meal out, but we don't quite fancy being in bed for the next two days. We would love to go for a walk, and even if we could with the fatigue and weakness, we know that means muscle pain tomorrow, and who knows how long that will last for.

I can say quite honestly that before I got sick, I used to take a lot for granted. Being able to up and go whenever I wanted, or pop to the shops. This is why the smallest things can make us happy. When you are living on such a low 'battery' you have to make difficult choices. As mentioned previously, any form of exertion can drain us. That means a phone call, looking through paperwork, or watching television can all leave us feeling terribly unwell. This is why we need to pace ourselves, if we don't then we crash. Crash? The M.E definition of crash basically means we have overdone it. If we say we are crashing then believe me we are not feeling well! The best way to describe a crash is to compare it to being fed poison. You can tell when one is on the way. It's different for everyone but for me my ears start becoming very sensitive to noise. The rustling of a crisp packet can make you cringe, and it seems like everyone is shouting. You begin to feel dizzy, sick and a headache comes on. Your eyes hurt just looking at things around you, and your whole body goes weak.

It doesn't matter where you are, you have to lay down. At this point anything we do is damaging our body, so when we crash we must stop everything we are doing. This 'softens the blow' but does not guarantee it won't get any worse. If we continue to do what we are doing, then it's a very rapid slippery slope. We feel worse and worse.

When I am crashing, as with many others, I need to get away from all stimuli. This includes television, talking, and light. The best place for us to be is in a darkened, quiet room.

There are lots of situations which can trigger a crash, and a big one aside exertion is stress. When we are stressed, our body goes into 'fight or flight' mode. It is often thought that people with M.E are permanently in that mode, and with the adrenal gland on 'high' – it drains the body immensely. I remember when I was first diagnosed and I had an argument with someone, I shortly felt as if I had been run over by a bus. So wiped out that even speaking was too much of an effort, every sound was too much to bear and I felt as though I had been injected with a poisonous substance. This is why we may distance ourselves from certain situations or people. It's that we cannot handle stress like a healthy person would – and even that's difficult to handle and has an impact on the body.

Another thing particularly draining is busy, noisy environments. I personally find this saps my energy very quickly! One of the hardest things is when people may see you for a particular occasion, and you may look 'well', but you've had to take it easy and rest in the days beforehand, and will spend the next few days recovering. People don't see that, and this is where it can be difficult for people to understand how ill we are. If they lived with us for a week, then they would see how debilitating the illness is. A good way to explain how we feel, is that it's like waking up with a hangover every day. Except we haven't had a drink the night before! You wake up with a headache, dehydrated, fatigued, heavy body and nausea, and dizziness that hits every time you move. Every single day. 365 days a year. Sometimes I don't know how I can feel so ill and still be alive!

4 HOW YOU CAN HELP

I often have friends saying they feel helpless and wish they could do something for me. Just them feeling that way shows me how much they support me. Sadly whilst you can't wave a magic wand, there are things you can do to help someone with M.E.

- Listen. Sometimes we just need someone to listen. Sometimes we don't need to hear anything back. We don't want to constantly talk about our illness but the reality is that it's a big part of our life and talking about it can sometimes help, a problem shared is a problem halved!

- Understand. If you are reading this book, then you may not have understood M.E, but by reading it shows you are willing to understand and learn, and that really is appreciated. Unfortunately there can be a lot of ignorance about 'invisible' illnesses but in this day and age, there is a wealth of information out there. So, if you are reading this, well done - you can be assured that it's one of the most helpful things you can do for us. And we want to say thank you.

- Understand our limits. If you feel frustrated that we are unable to do certain things, imagine how we feel! It's awful having to turn down invitations, or leave somewhere early, believe me it's incredibly frustrating for us when we want to do things, but our bodies simply don't allow us to. So please be patient, and don't take it personally. It's not that we don't <u>want</u> to do things – ask anyone with M.E what they want to do, and you will be given a long list! It's that we don't want to feel **more unwell** than we already do. Think back to when you last had the flu, I bet there were lots of things you would rather be doing, but couldn't.

- Don't talk about 'miracle' cures. If you can think of it, you can bet we've already tried it. All we want to do is get better, but the truth is currently there is no cure. If there was, we would be doing whatever it was, to get better.

- Understand that this is a physical illness. You can't tell it to 'pull itself together' – it won't. If only we 'got some fresh air' or 'exercise' then we would feel better, is not what we need to hear. Again if this helped, we would be doing it! Research proves that whilst exercise is helpful for some illnesses, it does the exact opposite for this one. It can make the condition much worse, be dangerous, and sometimes fatal.

- Don't tell us 'But you don't look ill!' – This can sometimes come across as accusatory even if meant in the nicest possible way. We may not look ill on the outside, but we can feel terribly unwell on the inside. There are lots of illnesses where people may not look ill, and in fact most illnesses are invisible. Arthritis, heart disease, cancer, MS, Lupus - to name a few.

- Please don't ask us 'Are you feeling better yet?'. Because if we were, we wouldn't be holed up at home or in bed when we could be enjoying life to the full. We wish we did just have a cold, and that in a couple of weeks we would be feeling back to normal again. The reality is that with this illness we don't know when, or even if, we will get better.

- Finally, please don't take our irritability personally. Feeling so ill every day grates on you, over time it wears you down, and at times it can make you feel as if you are going to break. Most of the time we try and ignore it, but at times it can get to us. If we are snappy and irritable, it's not personal. We simply aren't feeling well. Having these symptoms for weeks, months and years is enough to make even the calmest person snappy. Know that we are thankful for everything that you do.

5 M.E FACTS & QUOTES

- M.E is a multi-system disease, meaning all organs in the body are affected. This is why there is such a wide range of symptoms.
- In 2005, Sophia Mirza was the first person to have M.E recorded as an official cause of death.
- It is thought that Florence Nightingale had the illness, after she returned from the Crimean war. She was left housebound and too fatigued to walk.
- In 1955, there was an outbreak of M.E where almost 300 members of staff at a hospital were taken ill, and as a result the hospital had to be closed.
- M.E used to be nicknamed 'Yuppie Flu'. This is because it mainly affected high flyers, (bankers and city staff) and personally I think this very much supports the theory that stress is a predisposing factor to the illness.
- Over-exertion can cause damage to the heart, progression of the condition and even death.
- There is evidence to suggest that genetics can play a part in the likelihood of someone developing the disease.

Quotes from the medical profession and sufferers:

"ME/CFS is actually more debilitating than most other Medical problems in the world, including Patients undergoing Chemotherapy and HIV Patients (until about two weeks before death."
The Canadian ME/CFS Consensus

"I have had CFS for 25 years and am an 18-year survivor of bilateral breast cancer. To date, the CFS has been far more devastating and disabling than the cancer. Recently, our 32 year-old daughter was diagnosed with early stage breast cancer. Certainly, it was a blow to her and our family to discover she had a cancer in her body which could kill her. But I kept thinking. It could have been worse. She could have been diagnosed with a full-blown case of life-altering CFS, which could have affected her for the rest of her life. That would have been a fate worse than death for our high-energy, adventuresome, life-loving, and hard-working daughter. I mention the above because CFS is considered a "lesser" illness than breast cancer. Breast cancer certainly can kill you and CFS does not normally lead to death. But based on my experience with the two illnesses, I would choose for my daughter to take her chances with breast cancer rather than have to endure CFS."

An anonymous presentation to the CFSAC

"CAN you imagine not sleeping for 48 hours, then running a marathon with a hangover and a dose of flu? That's how it can feel to have ME."

Ceri Isfryn

"This illness is to fatigue what a nuclear bomb is to a match. It's an absurd mischaracterization."
Laura Hillenbrand, bestselling author of 'Seabiscuit'

"The whole idea that you can take a disease like this and exercise your way to health is foolishness. It is insane."
Dr Paul Cheney, Researcher and clinician

"My H.I.V patients for the most part are hale and hearty thanks to three decades of intense and excellent research and billions of dollars invested. Many of my CFS patients, on the other hand, are terribly ill and unable to work or participate in the care of their families.

I split my clinical time between the two illnesses, and I can tell you if I had to choose between the two illnesses, I would rather have HIV."
Dr Kilimas, Researcher and clinician.

6 THE M.E DICTIONARY

If you know someone with the illness, you are probably used to some of the terminology used. But just in case, here's a light hearted look at it.

'Crash' = A term used when a sufferer has done too much, and is experiencing an increase in symptoms.

'Brain Fog' = Used to describe the effects of cognitive difficulties, for example speaking, remembering or listening. "I'm quite foggy today"

'I don't feel well' = When we say this, then we are most definitely not in ship shape. We feel ill 24/7, so when we speak about it, we are definitely not feeling good whatsoever!

'I'm fine' = I feel like poo but I don't want to moan.

'I'm good' = I went out *and* cooked dinner today, without payback!

'I have a headache' = Please stop talking, my ears are very sensitive

'Thingy' = Used to describe anything we are too

brain-fogged to remember the word for. Surely you know what the 'thingy' is?

'I'm sorry but I don't feel well enough' = I'm sick to death by having to turn down things that I want to do, but am not well enough to do... this sucks! *Thinks you probably won't bother asking again*

And a few states you may see us in......

Pale face, slurring, dilated pupils – We have totally overdone it and are starting to crash.

Staring into space during a conversation – It's going in one ear and out the other... Why are you still talking?

Yawning – Please don't think we are rude or you are boring us, this happens a lot.

In bed, ear plugs in, eye mask on, in the dark – Yep, we've overdone it. Again.

Cringing when you are speaking – We know you are in fact barely whispering, but our sensitive ears are picking it up at the level of shouting, and it's unbearable!

REFERENCES & USEFUL CONTACTS

www.investinme.org
25% of all royalties are donated to Invest In ME, and independent charity campaigning for bio-medical research into the illness.

www.wiki.co.uk
www.hfme.org
www.supportme.co.uk
www.sophiaandme.org.uk
www.thegracecharityforme.org
www.ox.ac.uk

ABOUT THE AUTHOR

Hayley Green is an M.E sufferer based in the UK. Previous publications include **'101 Tips For Coping With M.E'** and **'Tickle ME – Stories of A Brain Fogged Girl'**

Printed in Great Britain
by Amazon

17631722R00020